Introduction to Archie's Story

Why Archie?

A brightly coloured knitted scar
Reminiscence Learning - many p   ascots
or dolls as a source of comfort   chieve
a person-centred approach to   well-
being for the person with deme

Red and yellow are the last col   d are
easily recognisable, perceived   rs.
These colours are therefore often used in decor   ome to
identify bedroom and bathroom doors, toilet seats, door-handles,
grab-rails etc.

Archie was named by a gentleman called Bill who was part of a
European research project called "Remembering Yesterday, Caring
Today", where people with dementia and their carers joined together
in reminiscence sessions and shared memories and stories together.
Every session Bill would greet Mr Scarecrow as he was previously
known, saying "Good morning Archie" before he settled down within
the group. He was familiar with the mascot and there was a sense of
continuity as it was always at each session. This in turn gave Bill a
feeling of safety and security, feeling confident that he was in the
right place. His long term memory prompted him to remember that he
had been in a state of well-being when he last attended the group
and so was more content.

Why write a story?

Dementia is a complex subject that can easily become too technical
and medical. So I decided to write a book that would simply, but
without being patronising, explain that there are many types of
dementia; the main signs and symptoms of Alzheimer's (the most
common type) and the fact that there is no cure. The book also
explains the things we should say and do to ensure a person with
dementia feels a meaningful part of their community, rather than
feeling ignored, invisible and unloved.

I used the idea of colour being drained from Archie when he felt in a
state of ill-being and feeling unloved and how the colour returned to
his clothes when he was in a state of well-being, loved and being
treated no differently from his friends.

Although the book was originally written for adults it occurred to me
that it could also be used for children to enable them to understand
the basic facts about dementia and how they could therefore relate
better to grandparents, parents or family members with dementia.
This would provide a satisfactory intergenerational link for both
parties and dispel the fear that is often present for younger people
and those with little knowledge.

Written by Fiona Mahoney
Illustrated by Peter Holmes

3

Colourful Archie Song

Archie the scarecrow was sad one day
His friends all decided that he couldn't play
His work was hard, his day was long
Everything he did just felt so wrong

Bland, dull Archie you look so sad
Bland, dull Archie bad, bad, bad
Bland, dull Archie you make such a fuss
Bland, dull Archie is invisible to us

His memory was going, he had lost his way
He started feeling frightened, his friends would say
Go away Archie, we don't want you around
You make us feel embarrassed so don't make a sound

Bland, dull Archie you look so sad
Bland, dull Archie bad, bad, bad
Bland, dull Archie you make such a fuss
Bland, dull Archie is invisible to us

His best friend Bernard knew something was wrong
Took him to the doctor to help him along
He explained about dementia and what he could do
Bernard told his friends and the farmer too

Bland, dull Archie you look so sad
Bland, dull Archie bad, bad, bad
Bland, dull Archie you make such a fuss
Bland, dull Archie is invisible to us

– 4 –

Archie feels much better his friends start to talk
The farmer asks him back to the field to work.
Bernard gives support and his friends treat him okay
No one is embarrassed just help him on his way.

Colourful Archie we love you so
Colourful Archie go, go, go
Colourful Archie you're the one
Colourful Archie he has lots of fun

His colour is returning and he is feeling good
He's started socialising with his friends like he should
Everyone included Archie in their plans
He feels more motivated and we all clap our hands

Colourful Archie we love you so
Colourful Archie go, go, go
Colourful Archie you're the one
Colourful Archie he has lots of fun

Invisible Archie is invisible no more
Everyone understands and they know the score
They don't ignore him or leave him out of games Archie
will never be invisible again

Colourful Archie we love you so
Colourful Archie go, go, go
Colourful Archie you're the one
Colourful Archie he has lots of fun

We all love Archie, we think that he is great
We know that his condition will only deteriorate
But we are his friends and always will be
However ill he gets he will keep his personality

Colourful Archie we love you so
Colourful Archie go, go, go
Colourful Archie you're the one
Colourful Archie he has lots of fun

– 5 –

Archie's Story

Let me introduce you to Archie the Scarecrow an amazing guy, one of the best and most respected Scarecrows in the community. He has many friends and works full time on a local farm. He has many years' experience and is good at his job.

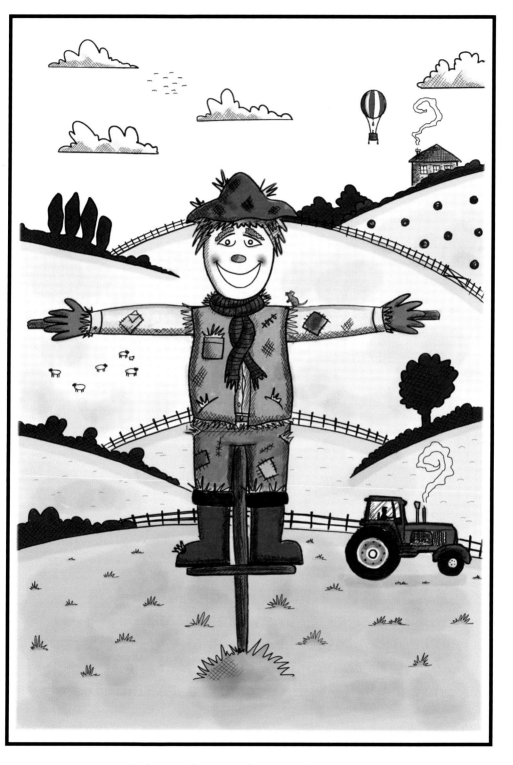

But recently he has become more confused and unable to communicate his needs. He is lacking in confidence and is feeling low in self-esteem and less motivated, plus his memory has started to fail him.

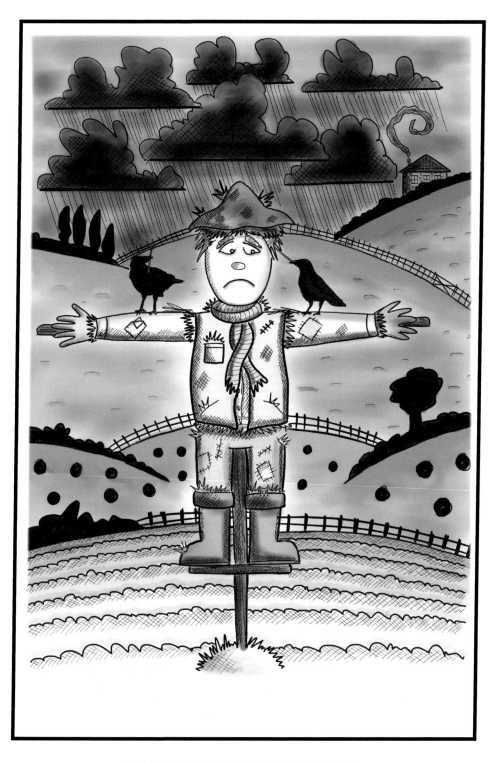

His job on the farm has become difficult and he often forgets what he is supposed to be doing or where he is going, and sometimes cannot recognise the farmer when he visits the field. The farmer is beginning to get angry with Archie and says he will have to move on and away from his farm if he cannot do his job properly. This frightens and worries Archie, causing him to permanently feel anxious and upset.

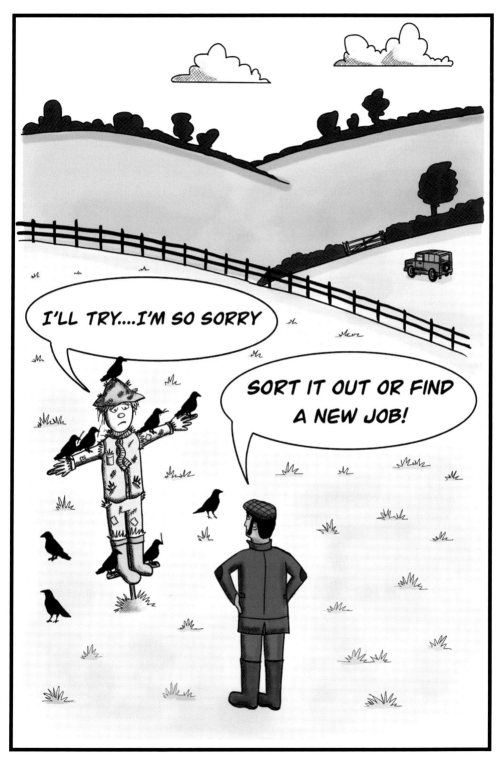

Occasionally when he talks to the other Scarecrows his words become jumbled which is very embarrassing.

Also he cannot always remember the sequence of how to get dressed in the morning. He has been known to put his jacket on before his shirt and regularly loses his hat. The other Scarecrows laugh at him and Archie knows they talk about him behind his back and this makes him feel sad.

At present he is still aware that something isn't quite right but he doesn't quite know what.

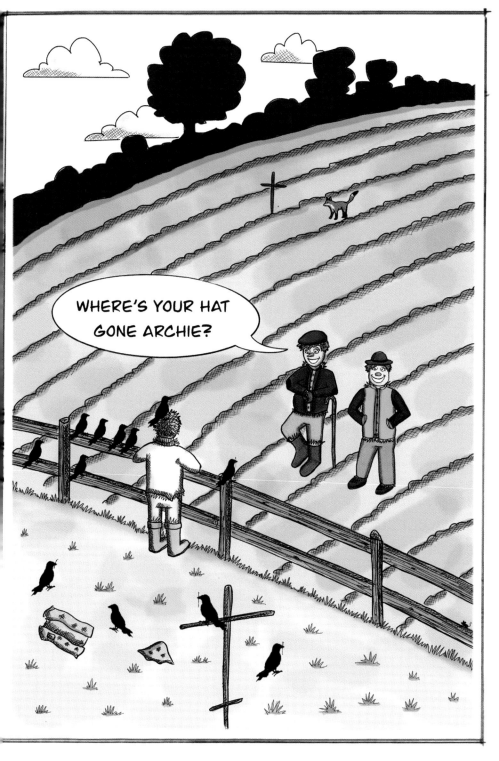

Archie's other Scarecrow friends start to avoid speaking to him because he is embarrassing them. At the end of a long shift in the field they often don't wait for him when they all go down to the pub and he is beginning to feel very left out and a little lonely.

Archie is beginning to feel his life is pointless and worthless. He feels as though all the colour has been drained from him and he feels bland and invisible to those around him.

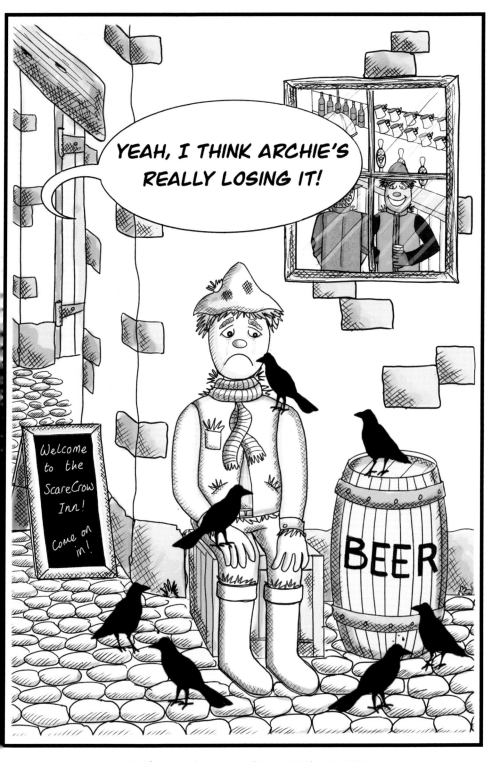

Archie has a very good friend Bernard who recognises there is a problem and decides to confront Archie about getting some help and advice.

Archie is a little worried by this but trusts his friend and feels a little uplifted by the kindness shown by Bernard.

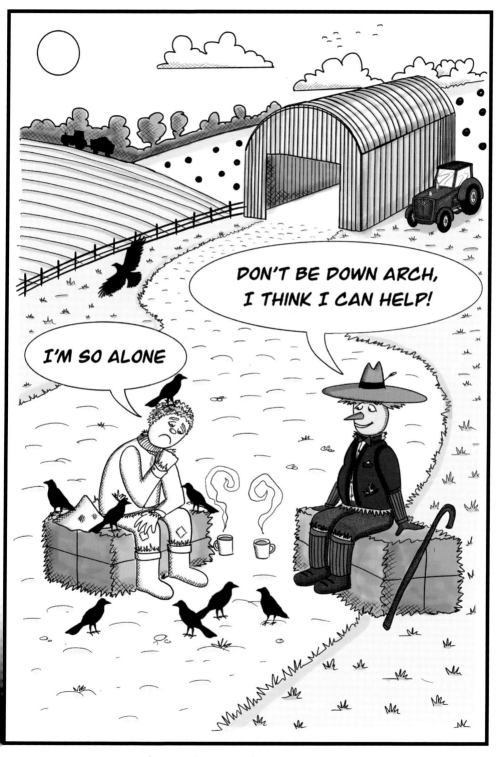

Together they visit the Doctor and discover Archie has Dementia. There are many types of Dementia but Archie has Alzheimer's which is why he is showing these symptoms and why his memory is so poor.

Archie is scared and upset but his friend Bernard looks up Alzheimer's on the internet and realises that even though there is no cure, there are things that can be done to help manage and improve the quality of life for his friend Archie.

There are some symptomatic medications that can help and lots of support groups and professionals who can answer any questions and provide the correct advice and guidance. He can even have a daily visit from a care support worker to help him get dressed and ready for his day on the farm.

Archie soon starts to feel a little more reassured and feels the colour is returning to his cheeks.

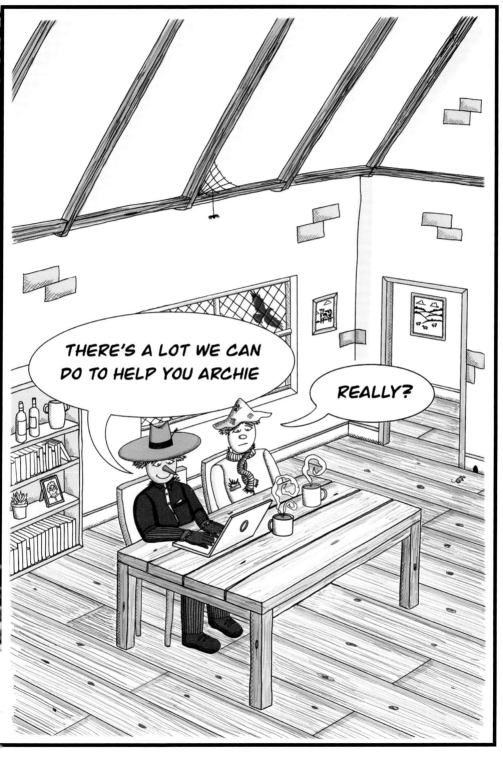

Bernard decides to speak to the farmer and the other Scarecrows in the community and explain why Archie has been looking so pale and out of sorts recently.

Soon they start to speak to Archie again and this gives Archie another reason to feel bright and cheerful.

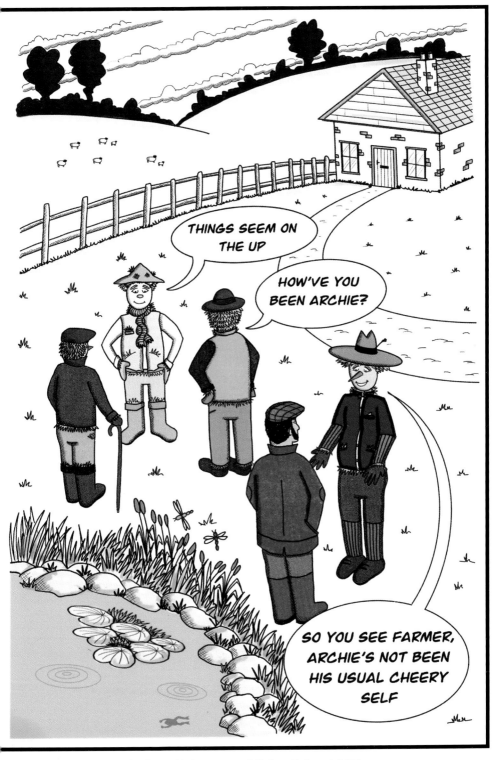

Archie hasn't been to work for some time because he felt invisible and unloved and had started to become more withdrawn. This in turn lowered his self-esteem and his motivation had reached rock bottom.

Bernard noticed he had stopped eating – sometimes because he had forgotten and sometimes because he was too sad.

But one day the farmer came to see Archie and suggested he returned to the field as a trial run to see how he got on. He reassured Archie that even if he still seemed to be invisible and the birds flocked around the bottom of his feet – not to worry he would put Bernard close by to help out if required.

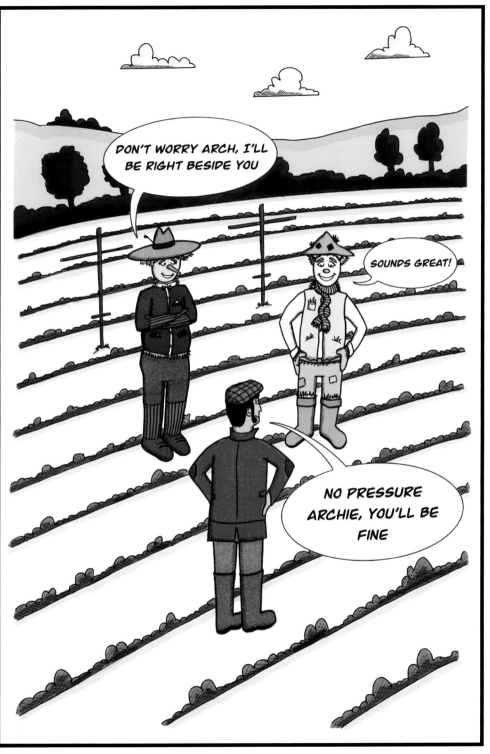

Archie started to feel wanted and loved again. Bernard helped him to dress in his best Scarecrow outfit and although it wasn't new it seemed to have a sort of brighter glow about it, as though the good feeling he was having inside was now shining through his clothes.

Archie had lost a little bit of weight and his clothes seemed a little bit larger than normal but he didn't care "Today is the start of a new me" he said, with a grin on his face.

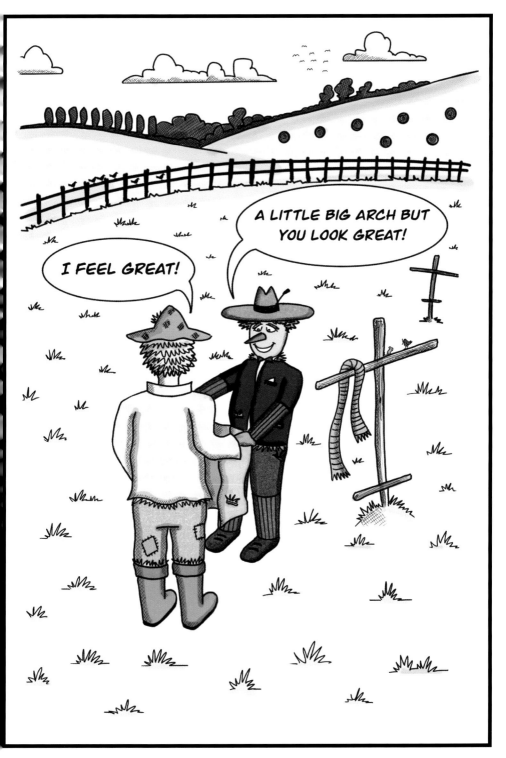

After their shift together, which had proved to be quite successful, Bernard decided to take Archie shopping to his favourite supermarket, to stock up on some food for Archie's empty cupboards.

They were both well known in this store and Bernard had spoken to the staff in advance to tell them that Archie had been diagnosed with Alzheimer's and although he was looking a little pale and thin he was still the same old Archie and not to treat him any differently than before.

He may be a little forgetful and say things that don't always make sense but he still loved his shopping and his coffee and cake in the café.

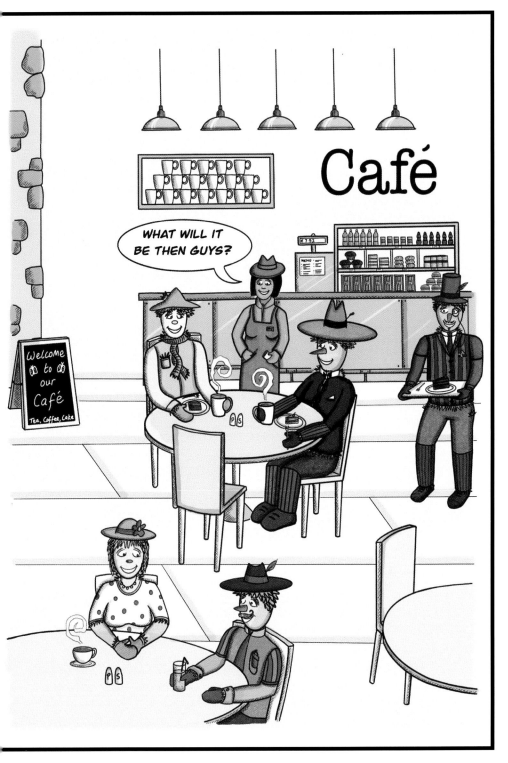

Bernard and Archie stocked up on all they needed – he even managed to buy a new outfit in a size that now fitted him.

All the staff chatted to Archie, not asking him direct questions and not looking embarrassed if they couldn't understand what Archie was saying. They just nodded, not lying but going along with his reality. Nobody patronised Archie or spoke down to him – he was just good old Archie.

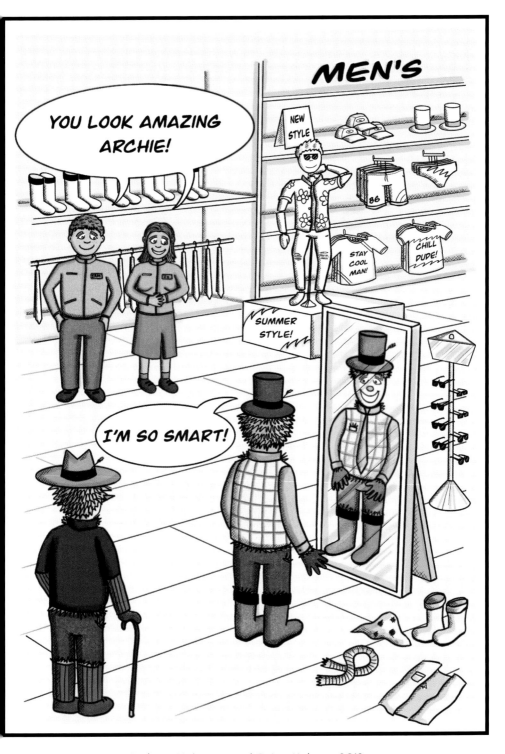

Even when Bernard went off to get some bread and Archie wandered off, talking about going home and looking anxious and lost, they just caught up with him at the front of the store and chatted to him whilst Bernard was told of his whereabouts.

Archie also decided to pick up some items and move them to other shelves but all the staff understood why Archie was doing this and just replaced the items without making a fuss once Archie and Bernard had moved to the checkouts.

Archie loved shopping and he was beginning to feel in a much better place and doing the job he enjoyed.

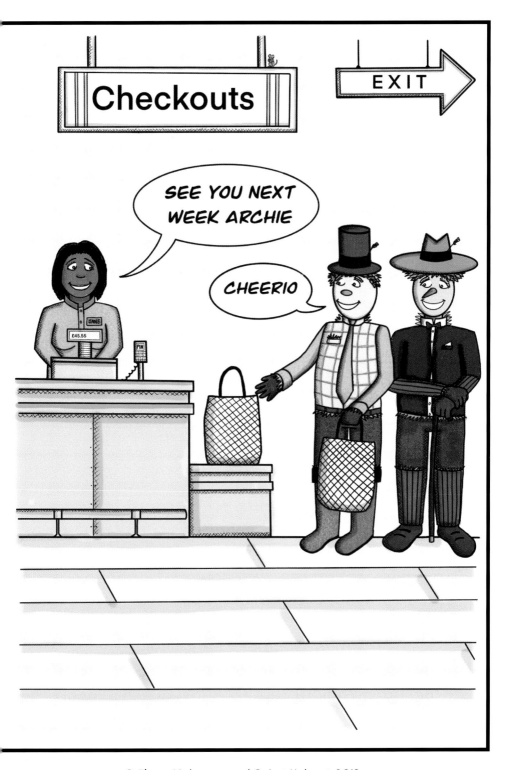

Bernard took Archie to another farm every other day where he met other Scarecrows with similar memory impairment.

So Archie started to make new friends and often took part in reminiscence activities about farms of yesteryear. He could talk about these stories and memories because although he had short-term memory problems Archie's long term memory was still intact.

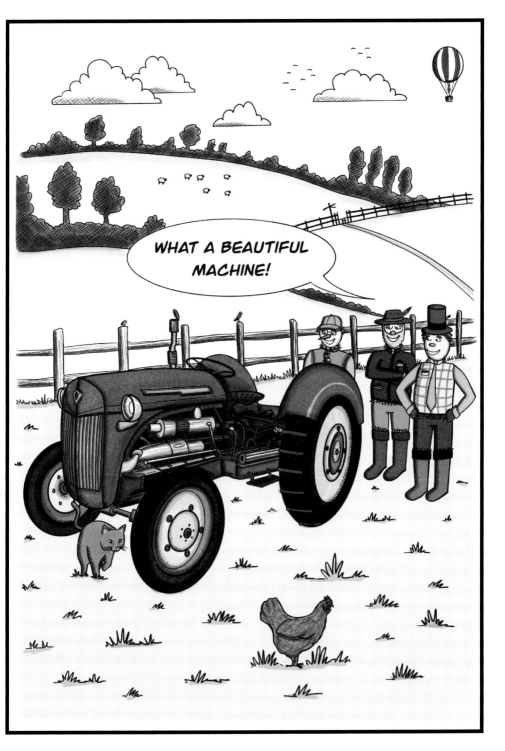

Over the next few months Archie's state of well-being had greatly improved. He looked brighter and more colourful. His friends were acting normal and even all the daily living activities were being experienced and carried out together with Bernard or one of the other Scarecrows – nobody was taking away Archie's role or deskilling him.

Although Archie was doing fewer shifts he was still invited to the pub afterwards.

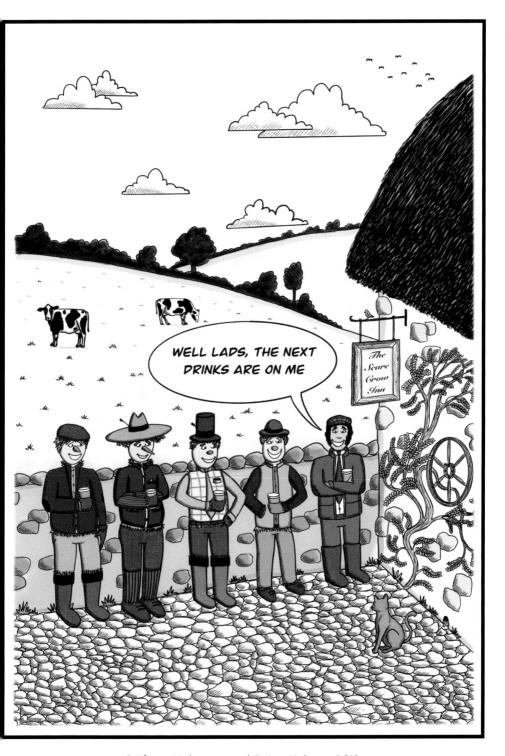

The more normal Archie was treated, the better he felt and the more colourful he became. Instead of being in a state of ill-being, he was definitely in a state of well-being. His self esteem and confidence had increased. He was more motivated and keen to join in activities and social events and he wanted to eat, shop and share good times with his best friend Bernard and his other mates.

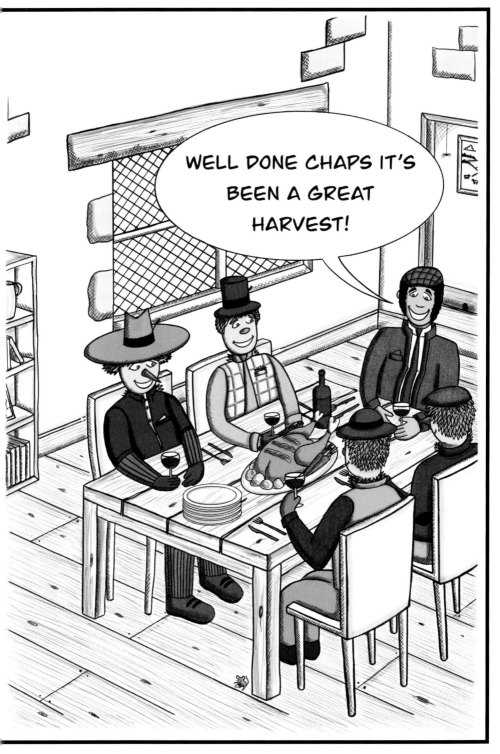

Bernard realised how easy it would be for Archie to start to lose his colourful personality again and quickly become invisible in the field and in the community.

He made a promise to himself that he would not become complacent about Archie's illness and although he realised things would only deteriorate and not get better, with the help of the farmer, his friends and himself he could help ensure that however ill Archie became he would never become invisible again.